# IMPROVES YOUR VISION NATURALLY THROUGH EXERCISES

# THAT WILL TAKE YOU 10 MINUTES A DAY

See better, exceptional sight, recover your eyesight and much more.

Ayuno Fitness

# Credits

# Table of Contents

# Introduction

Thank you for purchasing our book, congratulations on these exercises will help you improve your quality of vision, but we must be aware of how we use our eyes, the importance of taking care of visual health by correcting bad habits of daily life that directly or indirectly harm our eyes and our visual health.

When we spend a lot of time in front of the computer, we adopt bad postures like arching the back and pulling the neck forward, this posture what it does is block the arrival of blood and oxygen to the eyes, causing the extraocular muscles to tense and contract and that is when we start to have blurry vision.

The specialists insist that the blurred vision is not due to a physical defect of the eyes, but to the way in which we have learned to use them and that, if we manage to correct these bad habits, the vision will improve notably, for that reason in this book we are sharing to you exercises that are going to increase and to improve your quality of vision and to avoid that bad habits that consume your sight with exercises that you will be able to make 10 minutes a day.

# CHAPTER 1

## IMPROVE YOUR VISION NATURALLY

The eye exercises are millenary, they have existed in yoga for thousands of years, they are used by the great majority of people who are entirely dedicated to aviation, since they require to be continuously improving their visual quality because they need to see in perfect condition. In spite of this, the great majority of people consider the loss of visual acuity over the years to be normal, so much so that we consider it almost a common state that from the age of 50 onwards the average person has difficulty reading or seeing up close.

You have to understand the following, over time the extraocular muscles become rigid which makes it difficult for your eye to accommodate certain levels of depth whether you are nearsighted and have difficulty seeing at a distance, or presbyopia and have difficulty seeing up close.

There are many types of refractive errors that alter your visual quality, but for that there are 2 types of exercises that are very practical and that you can carry out in your life without any risk and without any cost, and that will cause over time an improvement in your visual quality.

1. It is the exercise of the muscles of the eyes, since when toning them and when relaxing them they increase greater range of movement, you allow the flexibility of those movements in himself and that facilitates the capacity of accommodation of your eye. This is useful for both near and far visual acuity deficit pathologies. Many of the pathologies are greatly benefited by these muscular exercises that we are going to show you next. The following is the aspect that has to do with the most neurological or neuroscientific part of the point.

What does all this mean? It means that you have a lobe in your head, the occipital lobe that is located in the back of your brain and is in charge of processing the visual information that we usually see.

There are a lot of corrections that occur from the time the image is displayed in your eyes until the brain processes it and finishes understanding it. Think about this, how an image that can normally be an improved photograph in software later like Photoshop, well your occipital lobe does something similar, so much so that there are many scientific studies that support as people with accommodation difficulties for example people with presbyopia, through training the brain to be able to perceive a higher level of contrast and a higher level of definition, not at the level of the eye, but at the level of subsequent information processing, increased their visual acuity despite the alterations in the rigidity of the lens and other pathologies that lead to visual acuity deficits in the eye that still existed.

Then we are going to treat the exercises the muscular exercises that allow you all that we spoke previously, as well as the exercises that have to do with the cerebral training that allows you to process the information better, to increase your level of quality and visual sharpness.

## EXERCISES FOR MUSCLE RELAXATION

1.MUSCLE EXERCISES: The first exercise is the muscular process; it is for a better blood supply to both the brain and the eyes and you will start by rotating your shoulders back and forth. Perform this exercise 10 times forward and 10 times backward.

# Forward Shoulder Rotation

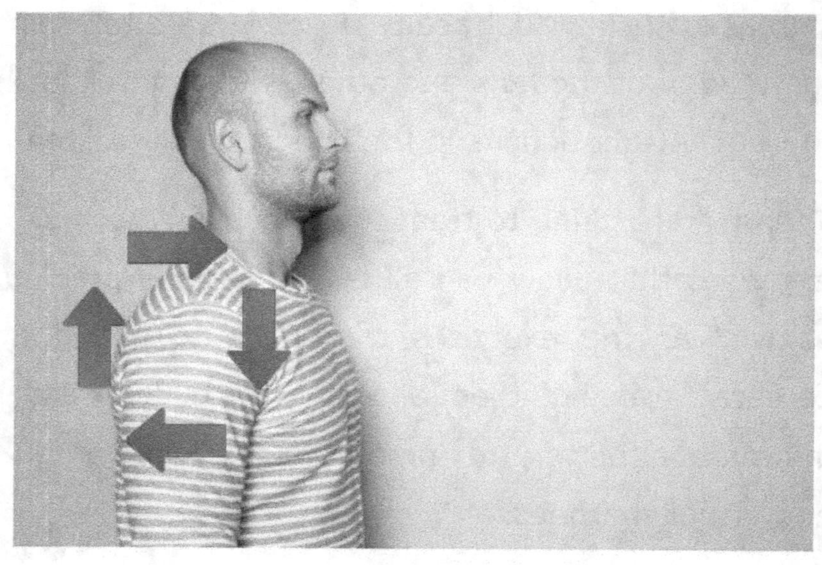

**Exercise this movement 10 times forward**

# Backward Shoulder Rotation

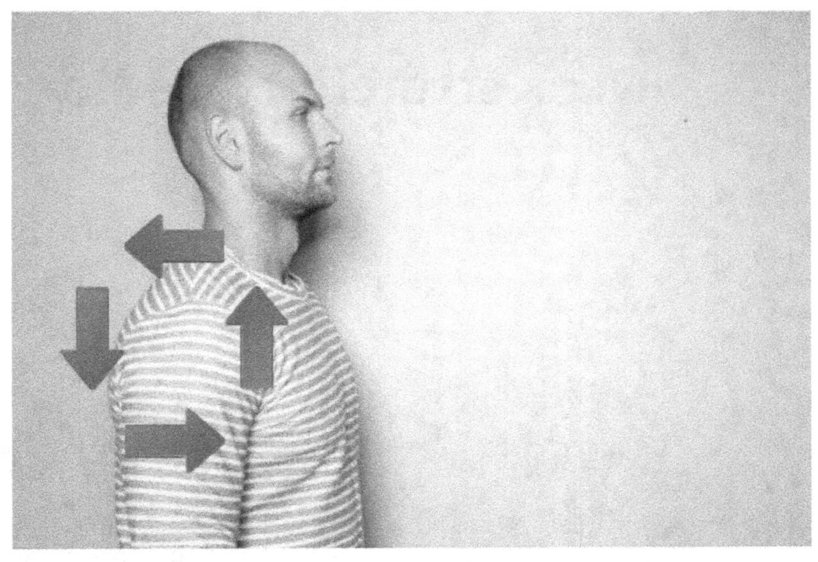

Exercise this movement 10 times backwards

2.    The following exercise will be used to relax the neck muscles to allow a better brain flow, you will carry your head sideways, 10 times (exhaling and inhaling) while you perform the movement.

# Neck stretch to the side

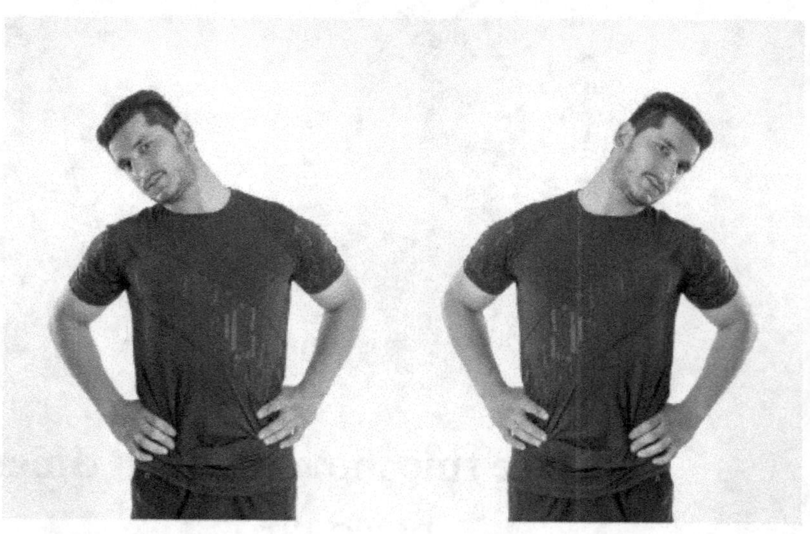

Exercise this movement 10 times for each side, inhaling and exhaling while exercising the movement

3.      Then you will turn your head circumferentially 6 times to the right side and 6 times to the left side.

# Circumferential head rotation

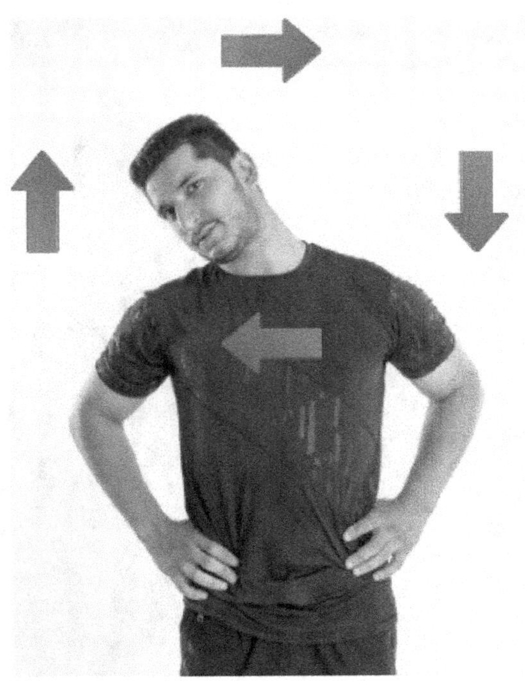

**Exercise this movement
6 times for the right side**

# Circumferential head rotation

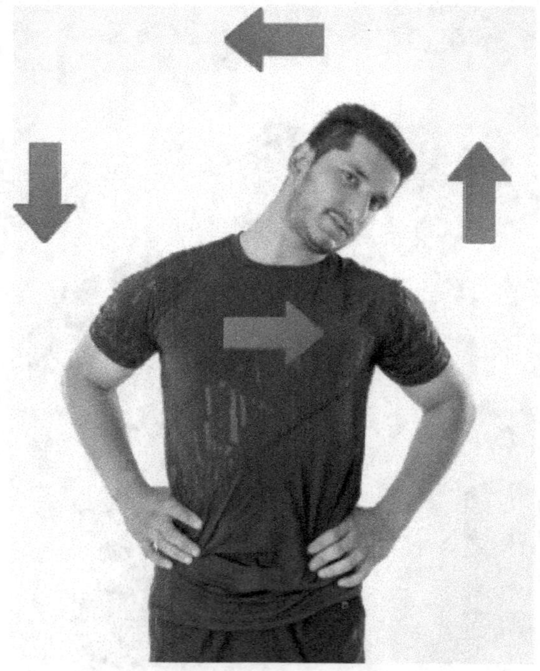

Exercise this movement
6 times for the left side

4.      Here begins the exercises for the eyes, you are going to begin to realize it with an exercise called palming that is to rub your hands generating heat and putting the palm of your hand on the orbit of the eye you are going to leave the palm 1 minute approximately above your eye, if it loses heat you can rub them again and apply again to the eye, to do it from 3 to 4 times.

# Exercise Palming

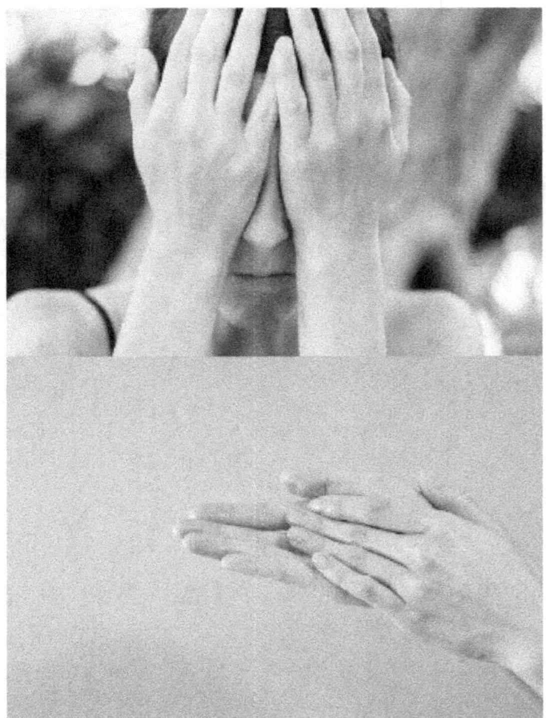

**Rub your hands together generating heat and apply the palm above your eye**

5.    Second exercise followed by this one is that you are going to begin to make a massage on the orbit of the eye and you are going to massage it in sense towards the needle of the clock, the tracing of the orbit of the eye covering with the palms of the hands. Do this exercise 3 to 4 times.

# Massaging the eye orbit

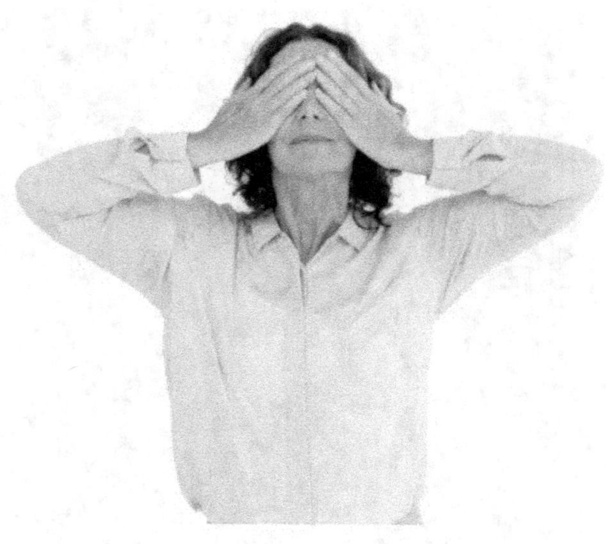

6.     Then you are going to take the eyes of lateral movements from side to side you can choose a point and take it from left to right and then from right to left while you inhale and exhale, keep in mind that the objective of this movement is to relax the muscles, so you do not have to force it when performing the movement. You will perform this movement 6 times for each side.

## Lateral eye movement

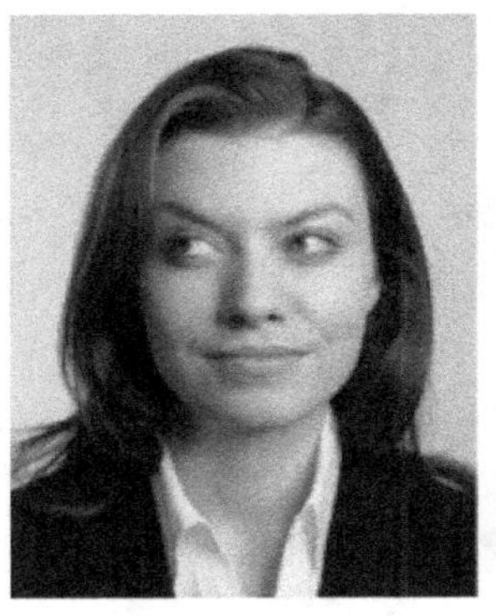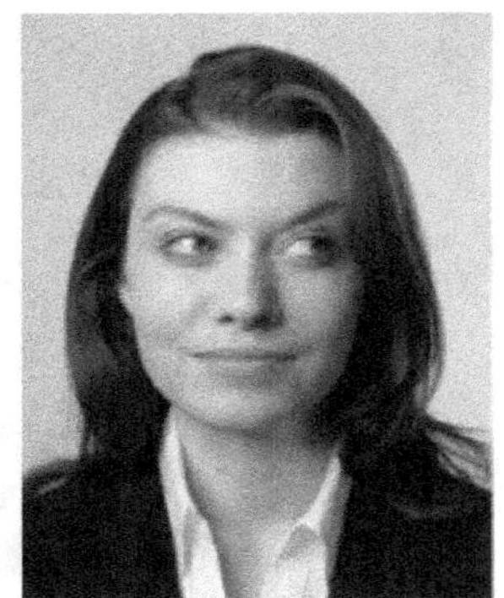

## Perform this exercise by moving the eye from side to side

7.　　Then you will perform this movement from top to bottom and from bottom to top, this type of movement you will use to make diagonal movements that start from bottom left and go up to the right and vice versa. Bear in mind that these exercises must be done while you are doing a relaxed inhalation and exhalation; do this exercise 6 times.

## Upper and lower eye movement

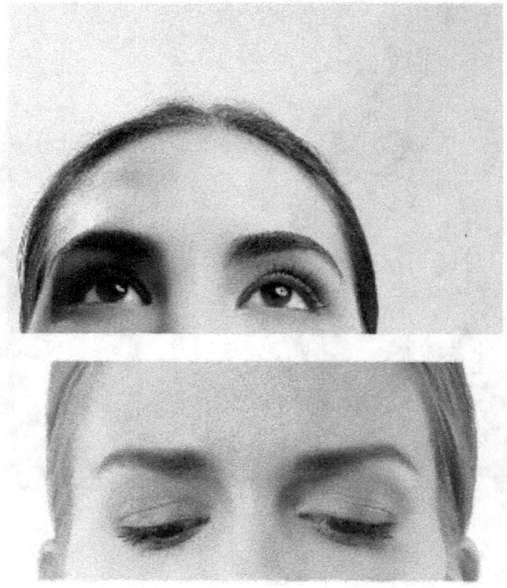

## Perform this exercise by moving your eyes up and down and diagonally

8.	Then we will perform a movement in which I turn my vision making a circle around my entire field of vision, this uses all the muscles of the eye at once and I may have trouble performing some specific section of the circle the movement. This is essential for you to notice which extraocular muscles in your case have a higher level of tension.

# Circumferential eye movement

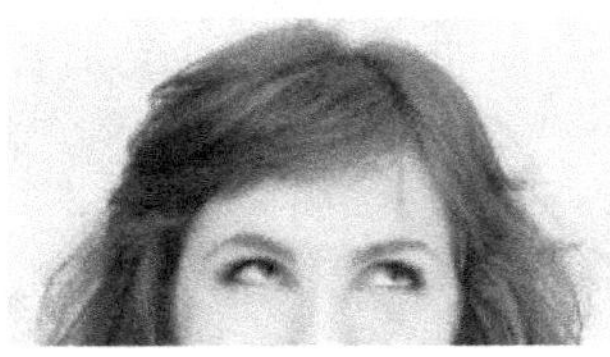
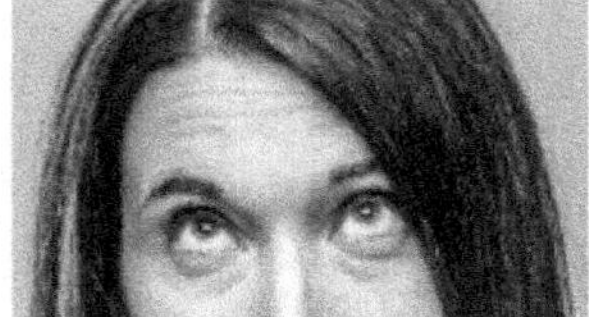
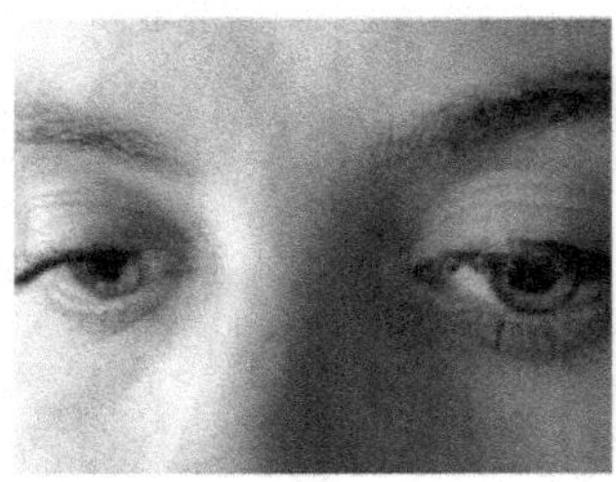
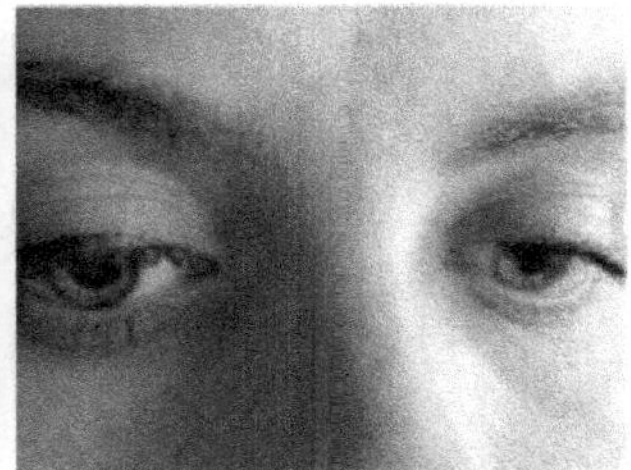

These were the muscle exercises, for the extraocular muscles, now we will see which exercises help the processing and visual accommodation and interpretation of that information by the occipital egg in the brain.

# CHAPTER 2

## 2. EXERCISES TO IMPROVE PROCESSING AND VISUAL COMFORT

1.     This exercise is called THE FOCUS CHANGE you will put your finger at 15 or 20 cm your finger, then an object that can be found at about 3 or 6 meters and an object at a greater distance to one that must exceed 6 meters and you will alternate in time from 10 to 15 seconds, the focus between a close object a medium distance object and a long-distance object, note that long distance is more than 6 meters for your visual ability, you will vary in the distance 6 times.

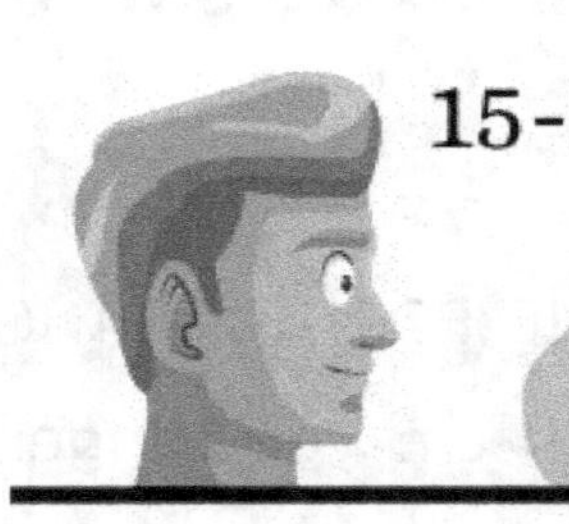
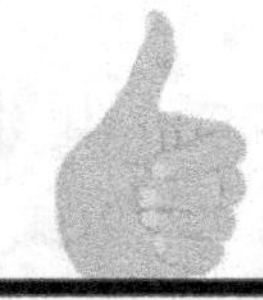



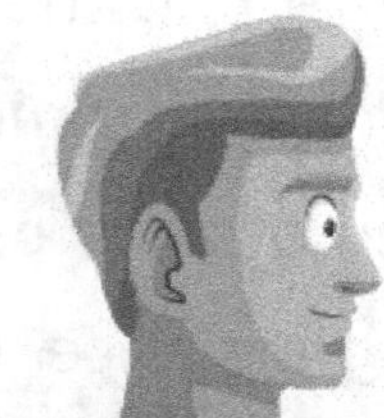
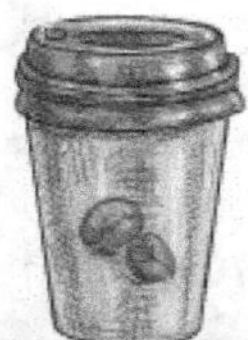



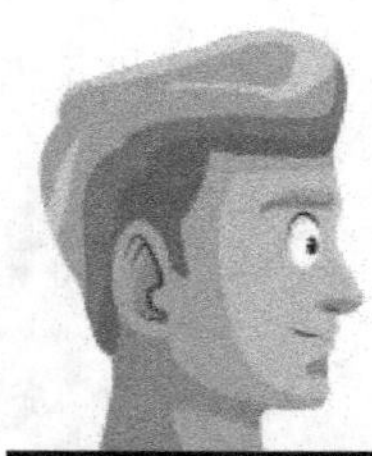

**Vary the distance 6 times**

2.     Then you will zoom in and out by training your finger focus capability at close range, from as far as you can hold your finger to as close as you can hold your finger without bending the image, always keeping in mind to inhale and exhale while zooming in and out.

## Zoom in and out

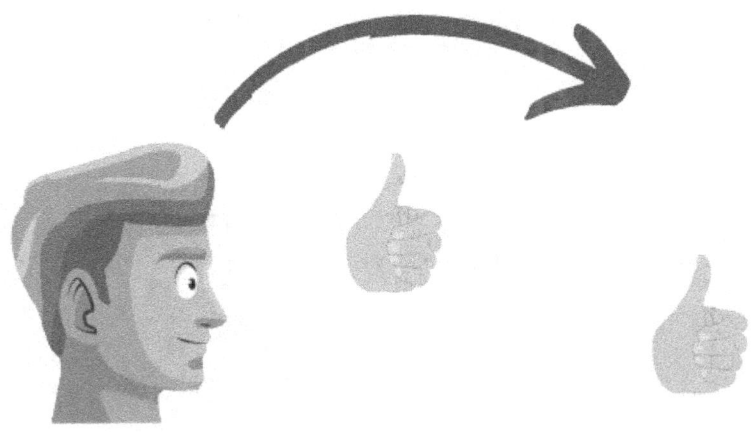

**inhale and exhale as you move your finger in and out**

3.    A very important movement for the visual coordination is the movement of the 8 or of the symbol of the infinite, to make this exercise in a vertical or horizontal way following an imaginary movement like the symbol of the infinite or the eight if you want to make it vertically, you are going to have many difficulties at the beginning to make this movement well, but it is normal, as long as you practice it in a continuous way it will be much easier for you to do it, and you will be able to exercise the route well, that helps to the coordination of the image.

# Visual coordination movement

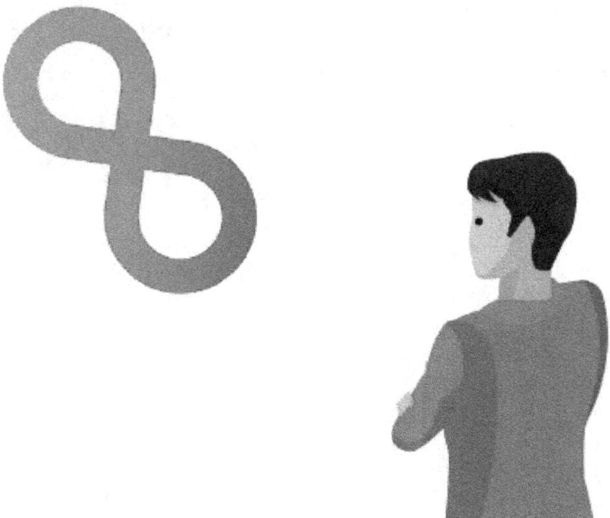

## 8 times vertical
## 8 times horizontal

4.     This exercise is crucial for those who have difficulty with near vision since it is the one that has been most scientifically proven and has provided the most beneficial results. In all people, whether you have difficulty with near vision or have cataracts, this exercise does not imply or generate a change in the muscles, but simply generates a change in the processing of information, making it easier for your eye to adapt to distinguish certain small images more clearly.

# Exercises for near vision

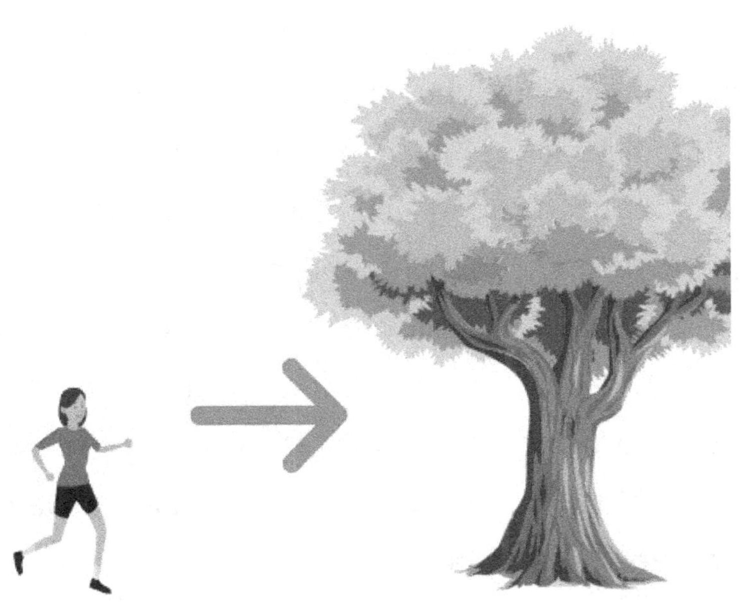

5. You are going to take a surface (bond sheet or cardboard) of a certain color that you choose, recommendable that it is black or gray so that it is more useful for your organism and you are going to put a point that is hardly distinguishable from the rest of the image and the color that exists in the background and you are going to try to manage to distinguish it by concentrating without forcing the sight concentrating in the point until you can distinguish it. If you have a near vision problem, you will get closer and closer to the cardboard only when you can easily distinguish the dot from the other dots. If your problem is far-sighted, you will do exactly the same thing, but moving the cardboard away as you improve your visual capacity. Don't get frustrated if it takes time, remember that all neurological skills are trained and this like all others must be trained and it takes days for your brain to respond to this improvement.

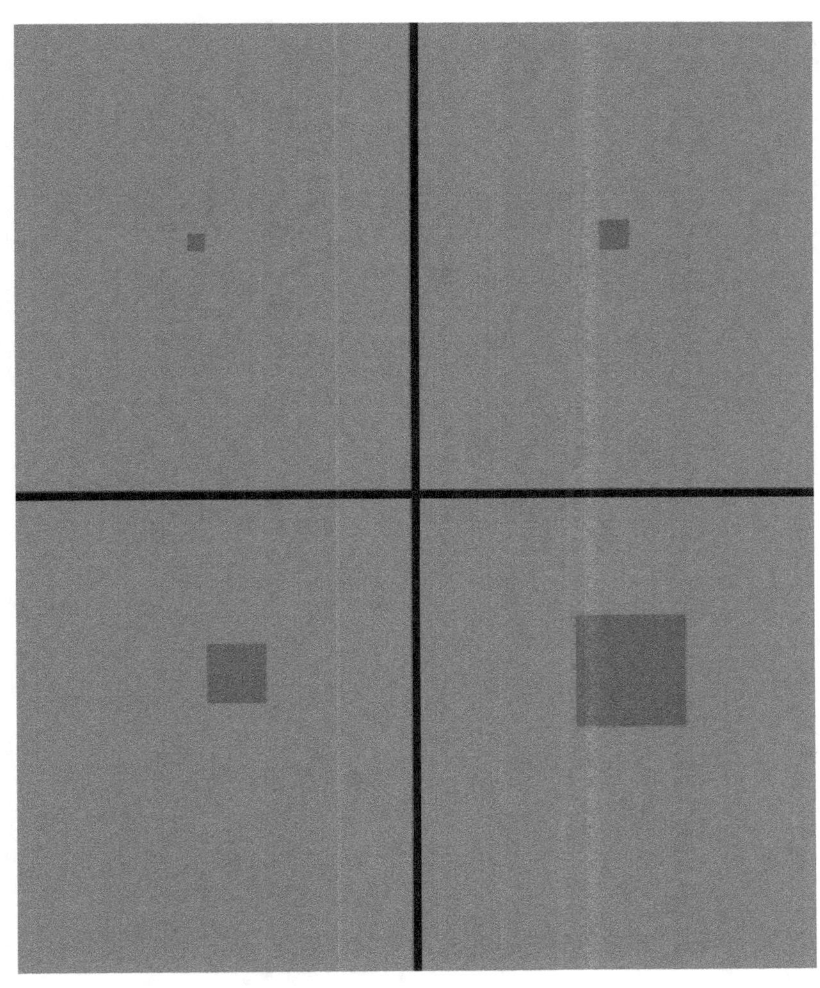

6.    Remember to finish your vision training with another clap as you did at the beginning.

# Exercise Palming

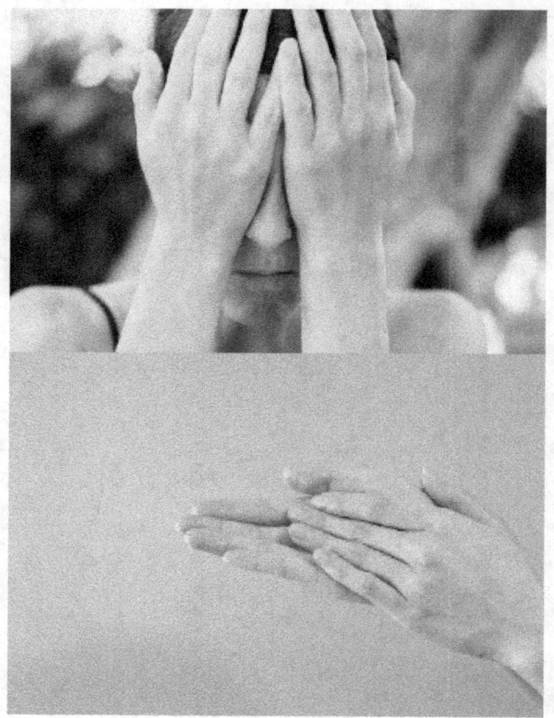

**Rub your hands together generating heat and apply the palm above your eye**

7.     FINAL TIP You can also use something that generates heat, you can be some heating gels or a bag of seeds or whatever produces controllable heat, to generate heat in the area of the orbits and eye sockets and generate more easily the relaxation of the extraocular muscles.

Keep in mind that you have to do this exercise every day and give it at least a few months to evaluate the result and see how good it is for your visual capacity.

Cure floating eyes here

# CHAPTER 3

## 10 TIPS TO TAKE CARE OF YOUR EYES AND IMPROVE YOUR VISION

These 10 habits should be followed to improve your quality of vision. Our eyesight is designed to see far away, but due to bad habits and abuse in many ways, we are losing a lot of quality of vision.

Now we will see habits that will improve your vision and that accompanied by the exercises seen before, your results will improve notably.

1. Perform outdoor activities, we spend less time in the open air and more time in small spaces, thus forcing our eyes more.

Before, children played a lot in the street, so the movement of the eyes was quite large and complete, now with mobile devices or tablets the movements that make the eyes are smaller, it would be advisable to combine with sports or outdoor activities and have a great movement of the eyes so that our muscles move in amplitude. It is demonstrated that people who spend time outdoors on all children have less risk of myopia less symptoms of visual impairment, so doing activities outdoors will help us to be able to improve our quality of vision. Keep in mind that if you work too much time on the computer or have a job in a closed environment, it would be advisable to give yourself time to combine with outdoor activities. Bioenergy and meditation here.

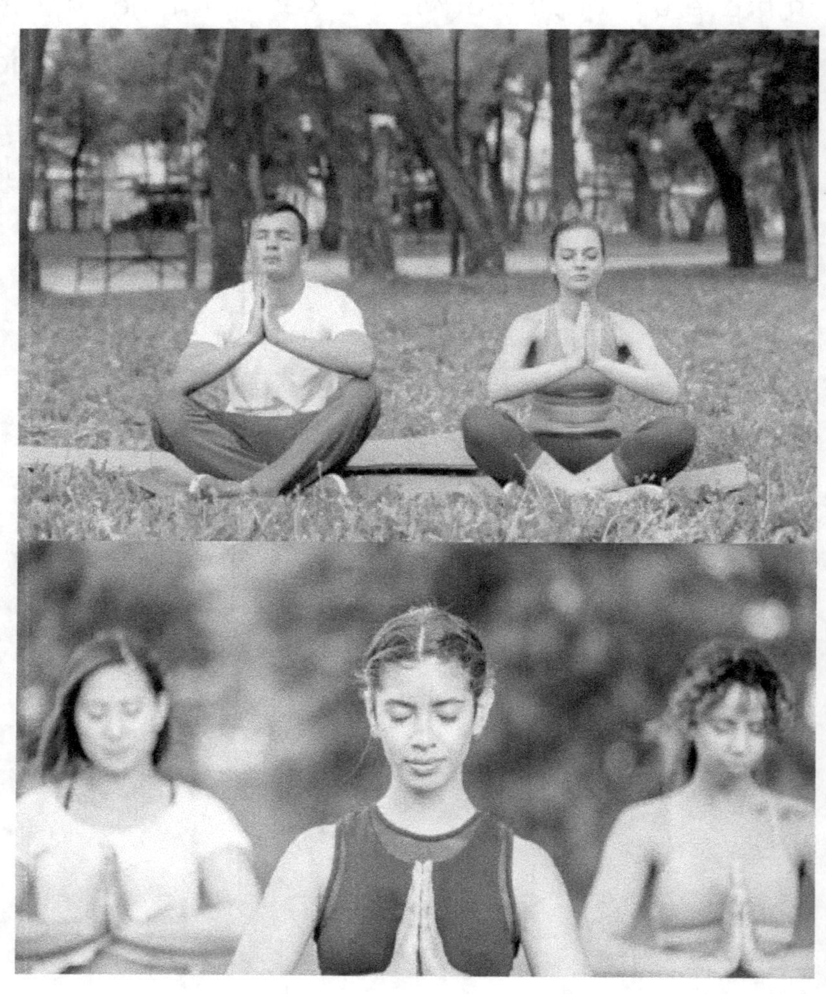

2.	Practice of ocular relaxation: although it seems strange some stretches for the sight, for the ocular relaxation, it is important before going to sleep if you have been a long time in front of the computer or in a closed environment it is recommended to do stretches for example to go out to the street and to see how many people pass from a balcony or to do exercises of movement of eyes help to that the muscles of the eyes do those stretches and the following day we do not wake up with a visual system whose musculature is a little seized.

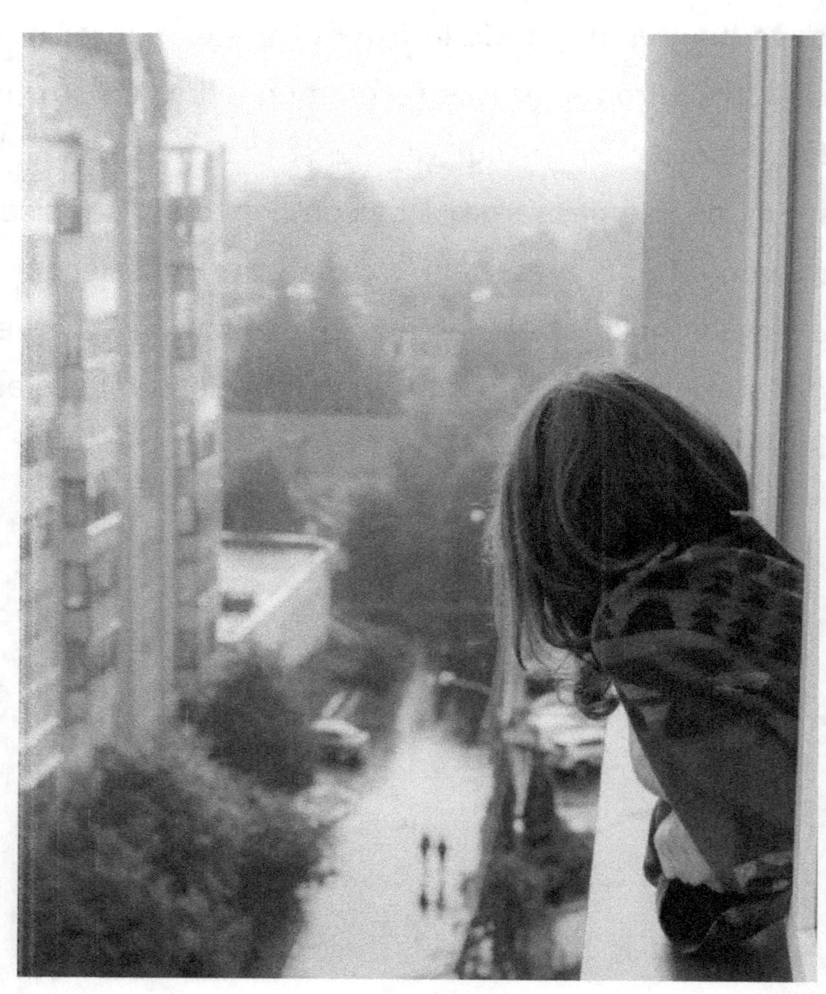

3.    Use approved sunglasses: protect your eyes properly from ultraviolet radiation, always use approved sunglasses, protect your sight when you go out in the daytime always wear a sunglass with high protection, even a polarized one improves the visual quality.

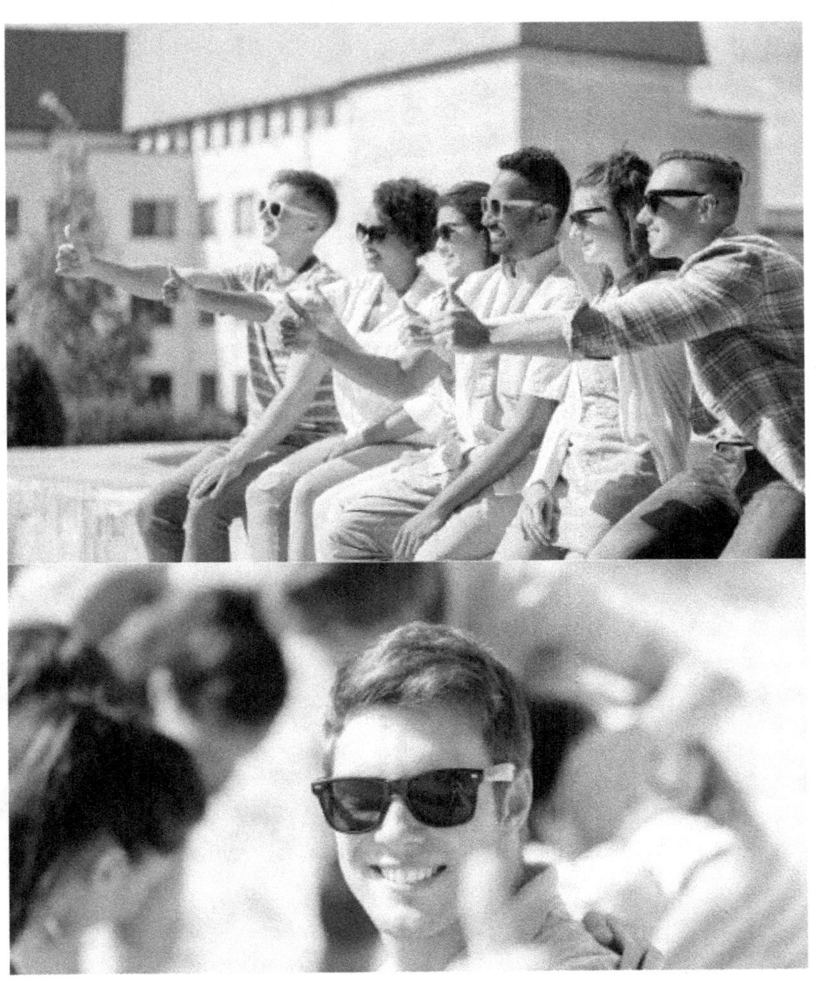

4.    Enjoy a healthy diet: did you know that there is an association between our food and our sight, eating healthy benefits our eyes, having a good hydration and a good diet consisting of fruit, vegetables, nuts, fish, lean meats are rich in macro and micro nutrients that help us improve our visual quality and also our physical well-being, when we are stronger our vision is healthier too.

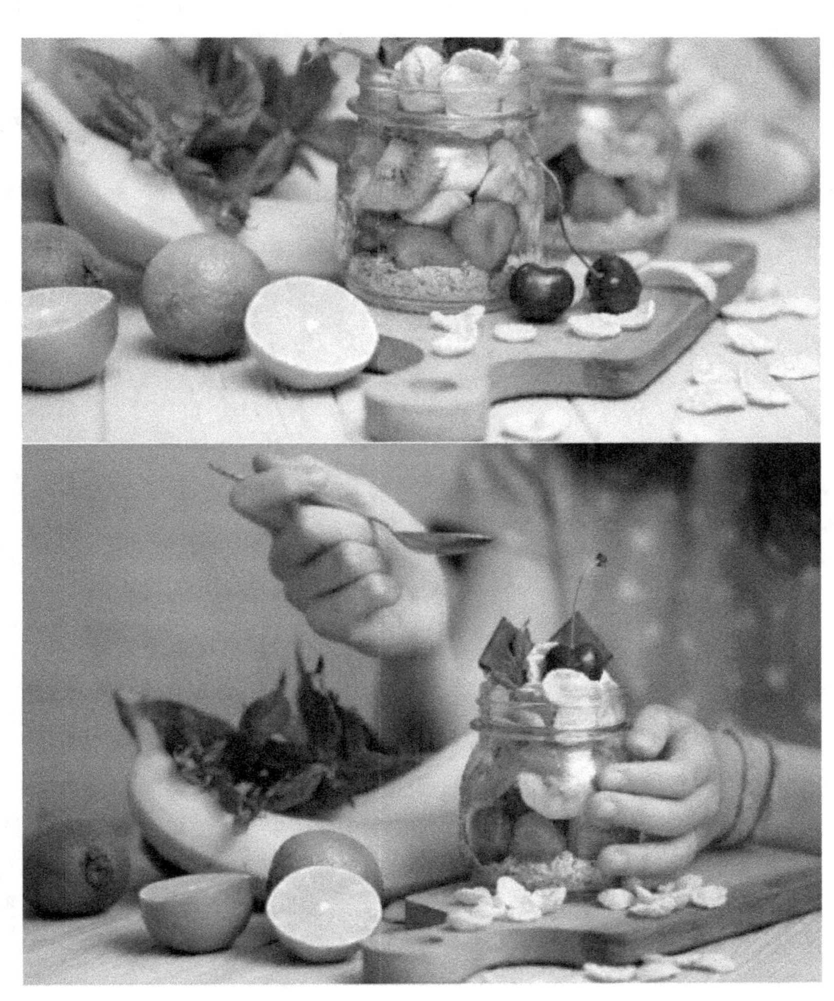

5.    Work with good light: this habit is as important as the others, it is to work always with good light, avoid badly illuminated places or in half-light, when you are going to read do it with a good light so that you do not make too much visual effort since you will develop more visual fatigue and it will be in a very constant way.

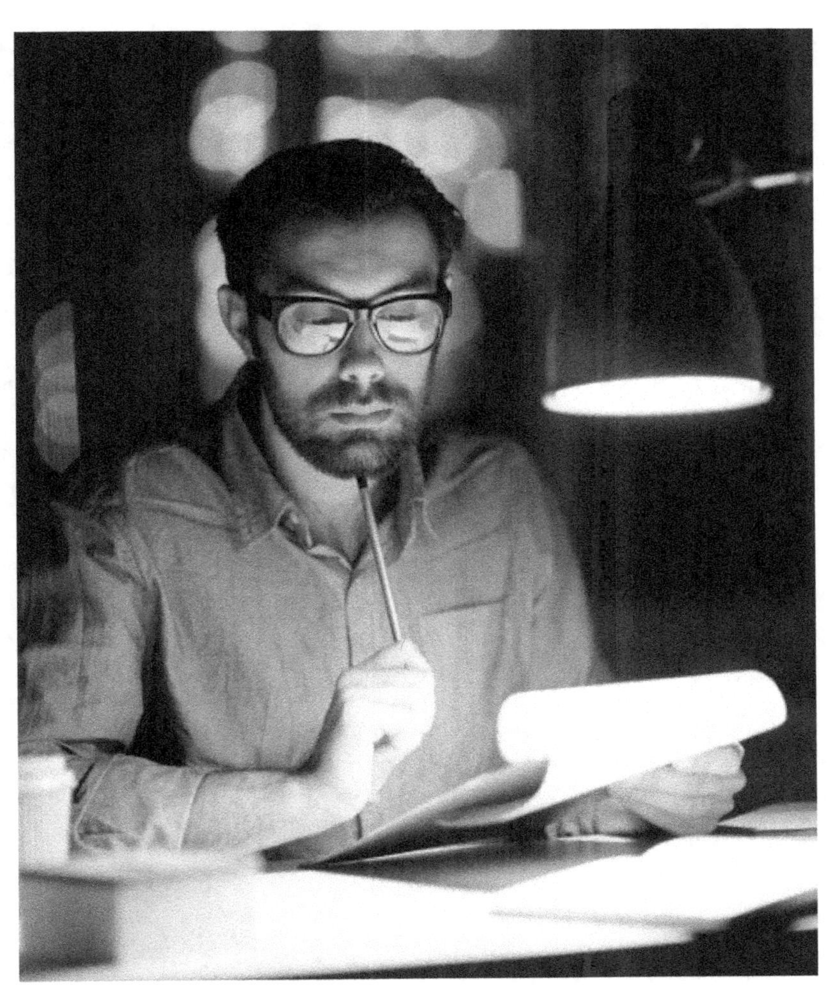

6.     Apply the rule 20 - 20 - 20: for people who work many hours on the computer there is a rule called 20 - 20 - 20 is every 20 minutes look 20 seconds at 20 meters, these are to relax the accommodation, within the eye we have a lens that is the lens that bulges to focus on nearby objects, this bulge must be relaxed so that it does not remain blocked in that position that would cause a pseudo myopia.

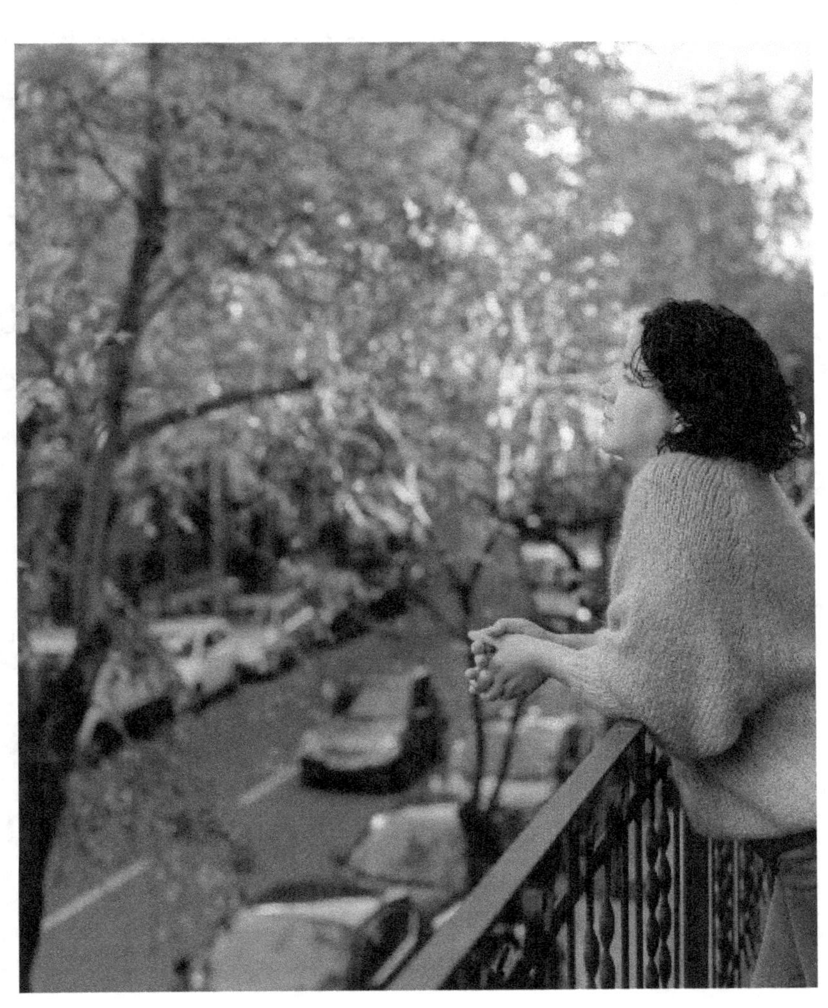

7.    Maintain a correct posture in front of the computer: you spend many hours a day in front of the computer, discover how making small changes in your habits will prevent you from having discomfort in your eyes, so keep your back straight, straight forward neck posture, because the neck is designed so that the cervical apophyses are not compressed backwards, the height of the screen is fundamental that it is halfway up the nose, that we can see on top of the screen, the screen slightly closer to the bottom of the monitor than the top, approximately 8 to 10 degrees of inclination and that it can be seen above the highest part of the computer, even if the wall is in front of us.

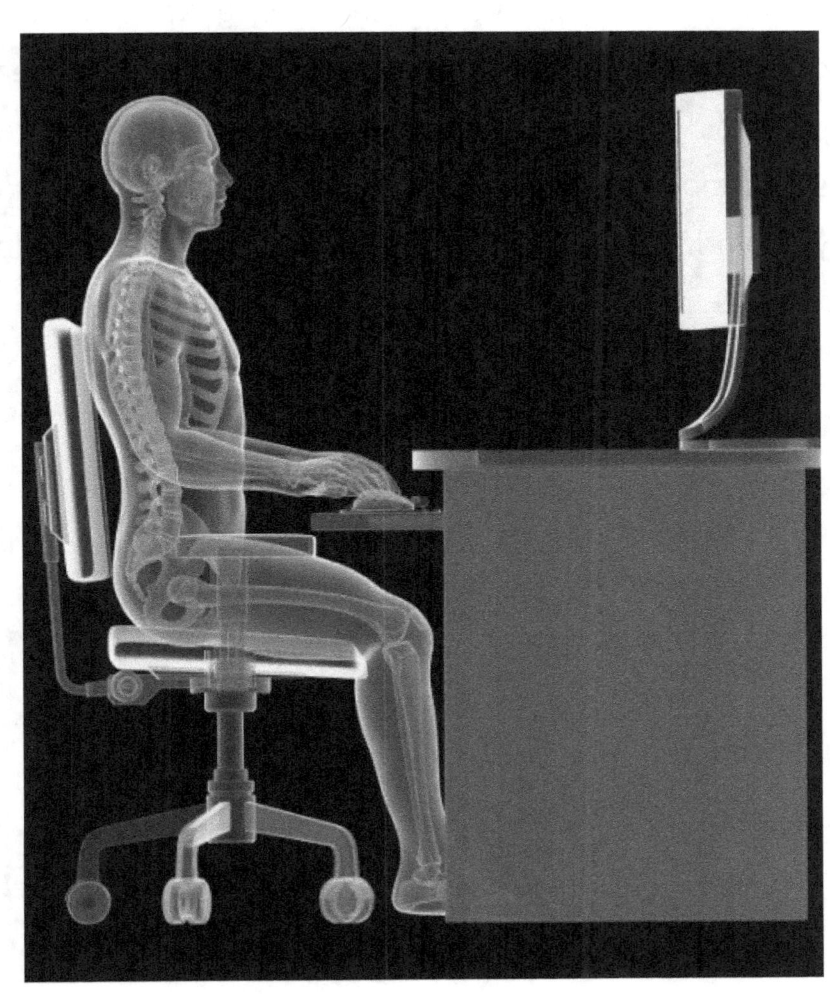

8.     Blink frequently: electronic devices today cause a decrease in blinking that must be avoided. To guarantee a good blink, approximately 15 to 20 blinks per minute, 1 blink every 4 seconds, guarantee at the beginning that there will be a good exchange of tears and avoid possible complications that today are very associated with the appearance of what is called dry eye syndrome, which is a fairly important problem today. Cure floating eyes here

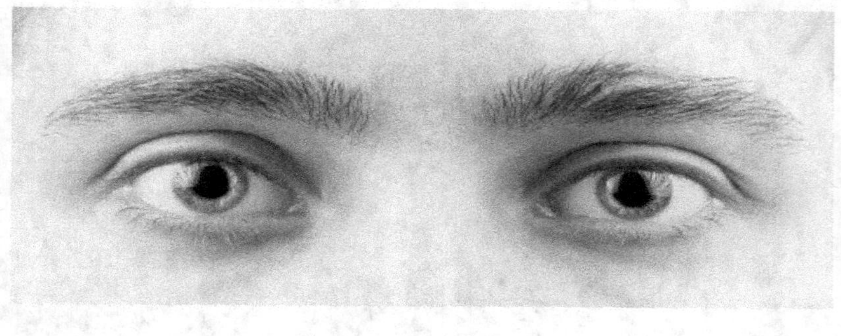

9.    Use the correct distance to read: the normal distance that is usually indicated is from the knuckle of the middle finger to the elbow, it would be to put the knuckle of the middle finger at eye level and that distance between your knuckle and the elbow is the most appropriate distance to avoid eye fatigue. If you could use a lectern it would be better, the lectern allows a distance of 50 to 60 centimeters that there is a lot of difference of accommodation to the 30 or 35 centimeters that we usually put the reading, then a lectern to about 50 centimeters makes that accommodation a little more relaxed. Now, with electronic devices, you can change it and increase the font size to compensate and not put a very small font size, those 10 to 15 centimeters of difference correspond to enough accommodation in the lens.

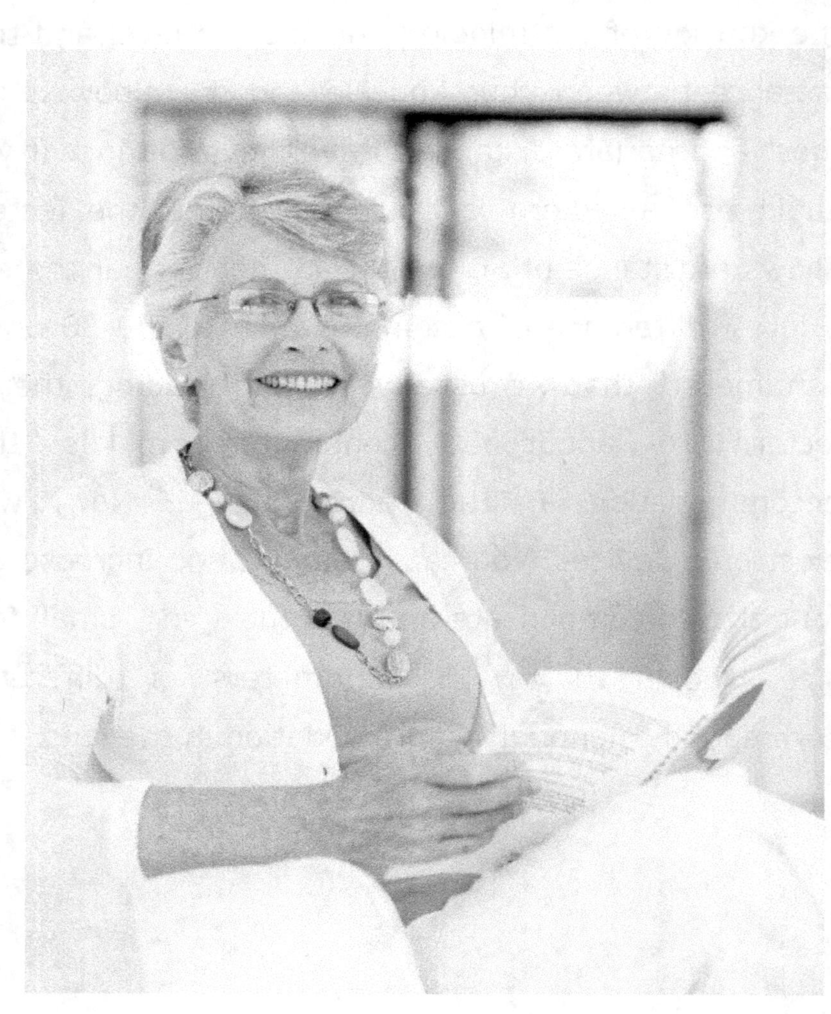

10.    Visit your optometrist every year: to finalize our recommendations of healthy habits you should not forget to visit your trusted optometrist every year to ensure better vision.

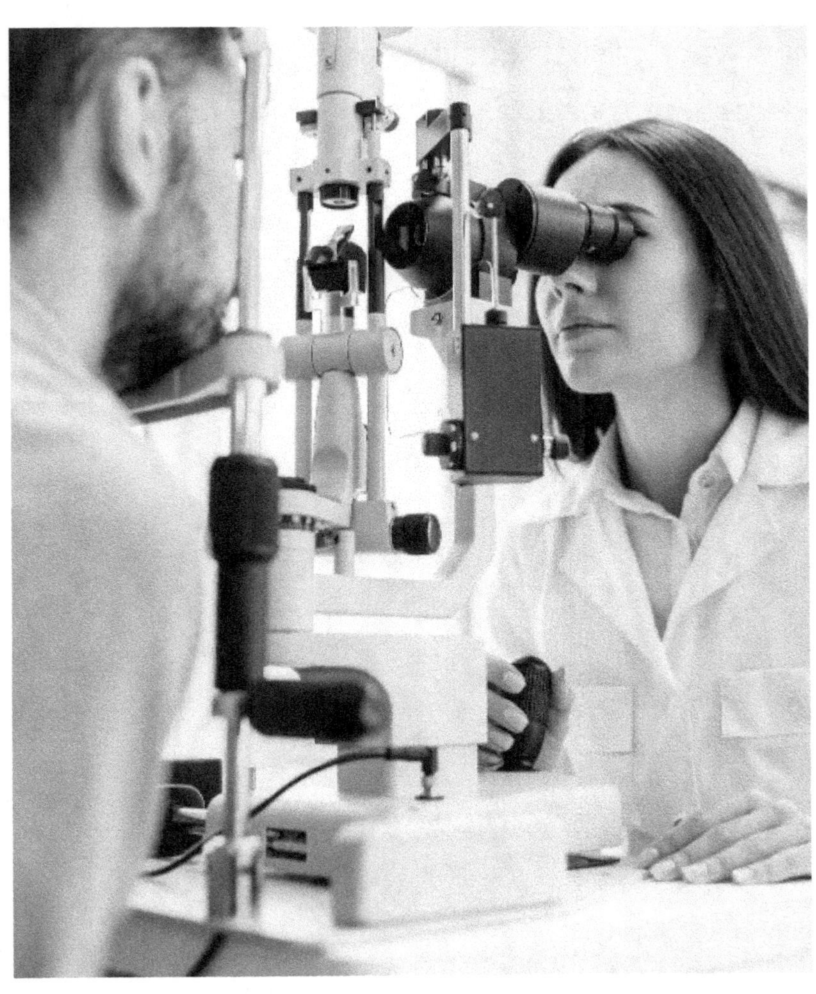

# Conclusion

We recommend that you apply these 10 healthy habits of vital importance in order to preserve a quality vision for many years.

Also apply the exercises mentioned above that will make your visual quality improve notably. Do not underestimate each exercise recommended here

9 798595 643054